DIETS TO HELP ARTHRITIS

A complete dietary programme to help all those suffering from osteo and rheumatoid arthritis.

By the same author
ARTHRITIS: HELP IN YOUR OWN HANDS
THE CHOLESTEROL CONTROL COOKBOOK
A MODERN BEE HERBAL (with Henry Rowsell)

Also in this series
DIETS TO HELP ACNE *Alan Moyle*
DIETS TO HELP BRONCHIAL TROUBLES *Alan Moyle*
DIETS TO HELP CATARRH *Alan Moyle*
DIETS TO HELP COLITIS *Joan Lay*
DIETS TO HELP CONSTIPATION *Alan Moyle*
DIETS TO HELP CONTROL CHOLESTEROL
                          Roger Newman Turner
DIETS TO HELP HAY FEVER AND ASTHMA
                          Roger Newman Turner
DIETS TO HELP HEART DISORDERS
                          Roger Newman Turner
DIETS TO HELP HYPERTENSION *Clifford Quick*
DIETS TO HELP KIDNEY DISORDERS *Harry Clements*
DIETS TO HELP PROSTATE TROUBLES *Harry Clements*

DIETS TO HELP
ARTHRITIS

by

HELEN MACFARLANE

THORSONS PUBLISHERS LIMITED
Wellingborough, Northamptonshire

First published 1979
Second Impression 1980

ISBN 0 7225 0411 X

Printed and bound in Great Britain by Weatherby Woolnough,
Wellingborough, Northamptonshire

CONTENTS

INTRODUCTION

One of the most persistent and long-standing theories in connection with arthritis is that the symptoms can be caused by an acid condition in the body and that this can be corrected by means of proper diet. In my own case, I have worked out a diet over the years which, along with occasional periods of physiotherapy and a sensible amount of physical exercise, has kept me free from pain and enabled me to live a normal life for the past fifteen years. Before taking these measures I had reached a point where I was almost ready for a wheelchair. I was also helped through prayer and meditation on the part of myself and others.

A detailed history of my recovery and the way it came about is described in my book *Arthritis, Help in Your Own Hands* (Thorsons). There is a sequel to this. Five years ago I became an enthusiastic vegetable grower, doing practically everything, with very little help and spending on average two or three hours daily in the garden throughout the growing season. The third year was a fairly dry one and I found myself having to carry water to the plants. Then the following year ushered in a serious drought, so severe that it became necessary to save water from baths and other household uses and make many journeys to and fro with buckets full – or nearly full – of water in order to salvage at least some of the thirsty vegetables.

All this proved too much for the right hip joint, the right leg being the one which for years had taken more stress than the other. By December 1977 it had almost completely broken down. A hip operation was arranged and this took place in March 1978, and I can only say that the effect at the time of writing (seven weeks following the operation) is like that of having a completely new leg. There was little pain or discomfort following the operation and this I attribute to the many prayers and healing thoughts which were sent out on my behalf and to the meditating which I myself have been doing for years, which would help to open the way for the healing to get through. Another very cogent reason for a rapid return to normal activities (though there was no more gardening) was the fact that a sensible, well-balanced diet has prevented me from putting on weight over the past fifteen years.

With arthritis every part and function of the body must be considered, as well as mental attitudes. It is not only a question of painful joints and muscles and weight control; it is also a question of viewing the body as a whole and realizing that arthritis is not a localized disease but a cry for help from the whole organism. In this context diet is all-important and no lasting improvement in any of the arthritic diseases can be expected if the sufferer concentrates on foods containing large proportions of white sugar and white flour and other devitalized carbohydrates, too much meat, cheese, cream, eggs, butter and frequent 'fry-ups'.

If the general guidelines in this book are followed over the long term the effect should be to reduce any excess weight and then to stabilize it to a healthy norm. This in itself will lessen stress and strain on weakened joints and on muscles and tendons which have lost their elasticity. Then, instead of a gradual and apparently inevitable loss of mobility, the way is open, if not to complete recovery, at least to improvement. This is a goal which can be aimed at day by day and the results can be surprising.

CHAPTER ONE

WHY ARTHRITIS?

Some of us seem to inherit, not arthritis itself, but a tendency towards it, and certain symptoms, which often develop early in life, are signposts pointing towards this susceptibility. One of these symptoms is chronic or intermittent catarrh.

Chronic Catarrh

From my own experience, backed up by my reading, I now realize that chronic catarrh can be one of the first symptoms of arthritis, and this is often accompanied by so-called growing pains. Apparently catarrh is one way in which the body is attempting to give warning and to throw off the poisons generated by excess food, or by a large proportion of the wrong kinds of food, such as white flour and white sugar products. Coffee and tea, except in moderation, are also bad. Ordinary table salt is another great culprit, since it produces extreme acidity. Two substitutes can be used for this (again with moderation) – sea salt or kelp (ground seaweed).

Vitamin A Deficiency

Another likely theory, in view of the tendency of arthritics to suffer from respiratory diseases in general, is that there is a deficiency of Vitamin A in the diet or in the system. This vitamin is found in the fish liver oils and in some vegetables. It has also been found that in many instances arthritics suffer from liver disorders, so that they are not able to transform the carotene in yellow vegetables into Vitamin A.

Assimilation of Carbohydrates

Many arthritics have difficulty also in assimilating carbohydrates, i.e., starches and sugars, and this process can be aided by the addition of plenty of the B vitamins, either in the diet (although this is almost an impossibility at the present time owing to food processing and other factors), or in the form of food supplements such as brewer's yeast tablets.

In fact, so important are the vitamins and minerals in sustaining health and movement, particularly for those suffering from arthritis, that a part of this book is given over to these substances and how best to obtain and use them.

Resting the Digestive System

Perhaps one of the simplest and best ways of helping to restore the body to maximum health is to make a point of having one day weekly without solid foods, eating only raw fruits or soups. This gives the digestive system an opportunity to rest and to eliminate accumulated wastes.

Any radical change of diet must be initiated very gradually. For instance, in the beginning meat could be omitted entirely for one or two days weekly, and in any case arthritics should not eat it more than once a day, and then in very small portions, as it is known to produce uric acid which is one of the main culprits in engendering and fostering arthritis. After a trial period meat could be alternated with other proteins, such as eggs, low fat cheese, nuts, beans, seeds – always in moderate quantities. These meat substitutes will be discussed further on in this book.

Avoiding Drugs

Another problem for many arthritics who have been on drugs for many months or years, including aspirin, is of course their side effects, and it would seem that the only way to get rid of these permanently is to get rid of the drugs themselves. This has to be done very gradually and even then there are apt to be intense reactions, including pain and mental depression. They must be tailed off very slowly, pill by pill and day by day, until the body becomes used to being deprived of them and is able to assimilate wholesome foods such as salads and raw fruits.

Perseverance

The first few weeks or even months of this new way of life, along with a sensible amount of physical activity, the gradual elimination of drugs and the working out of a diet designed to promote and restore health, may in the beginning produce unpleasant symptoms, as stated above, and will require much work and thought; but from personal experience I know that in the long run, if persevered with, it can bring countless dividends in health and happiness and a general sense of well-being, to say nothing of greatly increased mobility and a complete freedom from pain without recourse to drugs.

Like most worthwhile things these benefits do not come of themselves. They are there waiting for those who are willing to make the effort and to persevere regardless of the inevitable lapses and setbacks.

The more obstinate and long-standing cases of osteo arthritis might take six months or more to show any noticeable improvement, but improvement there is bound to be, particularly in general health, for anyone who has the patience and fortitude to study and abide by this or a similar corrective diet. Those with rheumatoid arthritis might also benefit from this regimen.

This is something each individual has to work out for himself, different as we are in our needs and abilities to assimilate the foods we take in. Trial and error must enter into this. There is an abundant variety of suitable foods, and a little thought and imagination can make any of them appetizing and attractive. This, or any other book or counsellor, can only set out guidelines.

Obesity

Obesity can be and often is a problem with arthritics and there seems little doubt that this can most often be the result of eating too many calories of 'empty' and useless foods, mainly refined carbohydrates. As Rose Elliot remarks, 'there are fat eating habits and thin eating habits', and these consist largely of the way food is eaten. I myself have observed when eating out that fat people generally choose fat-producing foods, then proceed to consume them very fast in large mouthfuls at a time. In contrast, most thin people take small mouthfuls, chew slowly and carefully, often talking a lot in between times. They are not concentrating on their food as if it were the last full meal they ever expected to eat in their lives.

CHAPTER TWO

BASIC NUTRITION FOR ARTHRITICS

Sir W. Arbuthnot Lane, one of Britain's greatest surgeons and nutritional experts, once wrote: 'There is no doubt that all forms of rheumatism are due to the disturbance of the acid-alkaline balance, and that this condition arises from faults in nutrition. Clinical experience has now amply proved that physical factors which predispose some people to rheumatism can only be successfully countered by a diet which puts all its emphasis upon alkaline-forming foods.'

Acid-forming Foods

Acid formation in the body can become excessive through the consuming of too great a proportion of the concentrated proteins in the diet. These acid-forming proteins are contained in foods such as meats, fish, eggs, cheese (except cottage cheese), dried beans and peas, and nuts. These should never be used in large quantities at a time and seldom more than once in any one day. For those with arthritis the bulk of the daily diet should consist of fruits and vegetables in one form or another, though occasional lapses should do no harm.

Neutralizers and Alkaline Foods

Strangely enough, the so-called 'acid' fruits, which include lemon and grapefruit, have a neutralizing effect on the body acids. In addition, they aid in the removal or dispersion of minerals which have formed deposits in the cartilage of the joints. Most fresh fruits, green vegetables and dried fruits have an alkaline reaction. Spinach and rhubarb, though known to be high in oxalic acid, are rich in iron.

I am setting out below foods which tend to be alkaline in effect, hence healthy for arthritics:

'Acid' fruits of all kinds, though gooseberries, strawberries and blackberries should not be eaten every day, even when in season; dried fruits, including dates are always good. Such vegetables as celery, watercress, parsley, mint and horse radish, tomatoes, lettuce, cabbage, carrots, preferably eaten raw in small quantities. Cooked green peas, brussels sprouts and broccoli are all good in rotation with one another. Spinach and rhubarb may be used occasionally.

Alfalfa in tablet form and molasses are both valuable foods.

A green leaf salad daily is most essential for arthritics, but those who have not accustomed themselves to eating raw foods should eat (literally) only a leaf or two to begin with. All raw food must be chewed thoroughly and slowly and this would be a problem for those with poor teeth. One weed which has been found to be particularly useful in combating both arthritis and migraine and other headaches is feverfew. Only a leaf or two daily is required in salads or sandwiches, but the beneficial effects do not begin to appear for at least four months. I am sure more will be heard of this in the very near future. Dandelions (the smooth round-leafed kind is the least bitter), chickweed, chives, mint, borage, and many other 'weeds' and herbs are also a pleasant and beneficial addition to most salads.

Vegetable Juices

Those who possess an electric juicing machine will have at hand a valuable tool for producing a good alkaline-reacting food from almost any fruit or vegetable, or a mixture of fruits *or* vegetables, not the two together. The fruits or vegetables are sliced into small pieces, then put through the machine with water added, and the resultant juice will contain all the minerals and vitamins of the fruits or vegetables with the roughage filtered out. However. this is strong stuff and to begin with only a few tablespoonsful daily should be taken, morning or night, gradually working up to a glassful. Yet food, as a general rule, should be eaten not drunk. Drinks are useful in illness or when fasting.

Use of Blender-Liquidizer with Raw Foods
This will overcome the problem of digesting raw green foods for those not accustomed to them, who have weak digestions, or have difficulty in chewing. It is also one way of using the coarse outer leaves or parts of spinach, cauliflower, lettuce, celery, cabbage or other green vegetables. These should first be washed and then chopped fairly finely with a knife or shredded by hand. The pieces are then pressed into the blender, never more than half way up, and water is added to about the quarter point or a little less.

This will be converted by the blender-liquidizer into a thick green *purée* composed of fine particles which are easily digested and can either be consumed as they are as a vegetable (though the taste is apt to be bitter), or added to a salad. Cottage cheese or salad dressing will disguise the strong flavour, or the *purée* can form the basis of a very nutritious soup. When milk is added the flavour becomes quite bland and further improvement can take place with the addition of a little kelp powder, sea salt, Marmite or other yeast spread, or soy sauce.

As in the case of raw vegetable juices, those unaccustomed to raw green foods should take only one or two tablespoonsful of this *purée* to begin with. The liquidizer-blender is also invaluable, of course, for many other kinds of soups, including those containing pulses such as dried beans or peas.

Other Uses of Vegetables
If a juicer or liquidizer-blender is not available, celery and the coarse leaves of vegetables can be cooked in a little water until soft, then squeezed out by hand. The resultant liquor is a healthful addition to soups, stews or gravies.

FOODS WHICH TEND TO BE ACID-FORMING

All meats, fish and cheeses (except cottage cheese)
These should be cut down to a minimum. The goal to aim at is to have any one of these only once daily and to avoid large helpings at any time.

Eggs and Egg Products
No more than the equivalent of two or three eggs should be eaten weekly. Eggs are more easily assimilated when mixed with milk, as when scrambled.

Dried Beans, including Lentils, Dried Peas and Nuts
These could be alternated with flesh foods, cheese and eggs for protein and never used in large quantities at any one time.

All White Sugar and White Flour Products
These should be used only occasionally and then sparingly on special occasions.

Alcoholic Drinks
With the possible exception of good wines (not sherry) these should not be consumed daily and never in large amounts at a time.

Deep Fried Foods
Should never be eaten.

Strong Tea and Strong Coffee
If used several times a day these can be harmful, particularly to the kidneys and the liver. They are acid-producing and are likely to increase the arthritic symptoms.

Other harmful substances are salt (except sea salt in moderation), pickles, most sauces.

The following is an excerpt from the writings of Dr Howard Hay: 'There is no such thing as an incurable case of arthritis, although damage done to the joints previously by years of arthritis may never be fully corrected. The process, however, can be halted and a great deal of improvement enjoyed in every case ... I would not touch starch or sugar in any form, but would live entirely on cooked vegetables, raw vegetable salads, fresh fruit and milk or buttermilk and cheese. In addition, I would suggest that you get a preparation of wheatgerm and take a tablespoon of this three times a day with honey ... '

Thr Through my own experience with arthritis I find myself disagreeing with Dr Hay in some respects. For instance I believe that a moderate amount of meat or fish once daily is preferable to consuming large quantities of milk products, including cheese, which are liable to lead to catarrh or to increase any bronchial tendencies. However, it must always be borne in mind that no two individuals are alike in their nutritional requirements and that no so-called authority can do any more than lay down general guidelines. Only through observation, trial and error over a fairly long period of time can anyone work out the diet which will bring him the maximum degree of health.

Set-backs

Dr Hay continues: 'It is not unusual to have a marked aggravation of the arthritis after you first begin changing the body's chemistry, and this is caused not by anything you are eating, but by chemicals already stored in your body that are still being precipitated. Go on in this way for a number of weeks, and you will find the condition arrested, for the pain is less and the attacks of acute arthritis less frequent and less severe.'

It is known that these apparent set-backs are all part of the healing process and a sign that the body is responding. Very often a day on vegetable soup or mild fruits such as grapes or apples will put things right again. One bonus of a diet containing plenty of fresh fruits and vegetables is that they are known to enrich the blood stream, which in turn could lead to an improvement in circulation. Poor circulation is generally associated with rheumatism and arthritis and could be one of the contributory causes.

CHAPTER THREE

OTHER NUTRITIONAL GUIDELINES

Broadly speaking, to function well the body requires proteins, fats, carbohydrates, minerals, vitamins, and various trace elements. At one time all of these and other essential elements would have been present in an ordinary 'well-balanced' diet, but the methods used today to produce, refine and/or process our foods have destroyed many (if not all in some instances) of the life-giving constituents formerly present in our diet. To replace at least some of these it has become almost a necessity to use food supplements, which will be the subject of another chapter.

Proteins
The amount of protein required each day per person has long been in dispute, but some of the best authorities have now come round to the view that the tendency in the developed countries has been to use quantities far in excess of the requirements of the body. This would particularly be the case for arthritics, since nearly all proteins, whether of animal or vegetable origin, are acid-producing, with the possible exception of the green-leaf proteins. Therefore the safest and best course is to limit the consumption of meat to one small portion daily, as previously stated, and when using vegetable proteins such as beans, again to take very little at a time. The same caution should be used with eggs, cheese, and other dairy products. Nuts and seeds are other good sources of protein, but here again care should be taken as to quantity.

It has now been recognized by some of those who have delved deeply into the field (not yet a 'science') of nutrition that green-leaf and whole grain proteins can be rated as valuable foods, particularly if they are properly combined with other proteins so that 'complete' usable protein results. This will be explained in more detail in Chapter Five.

Fats
Anything relating to the consumption of fats is at present an extremely controversial subject about which hardly any two 'authorities' will agree. The only safe rule for anyone is to eat only the lean parts of meat, to avoid deep-fried foods of all kinds, to avoid lard, pastries and rich puddings, to use limited quantities of butter and cream and to concentrate on the margarines which claim to be 'cholesterol-free'. However, even some of these may be suspect because of the processing methods used in their manufacture. Moderate quantities again must be the answer to this problem.

One reason why arthritics should try to avoid the build-up of cholesterol in their veins and arteries is not only to decrease the possibility of coronaries or strokes but because this build-up will inhibit the circulation of the blood, which could be in itself one of the causes of arthritis, particularly when the muscles are affected.

Although it is as well to avoid certain fats and to consume others in limited quantities, investigators have discovered that in many primitive societies people can use large quantities of animal fats daily yet remain free from excess cholesterol until they begin to include in their diet relatively large proportions of 'civilized' food, i.e., white sugar, white flour and other devitalized carbohydrates.

Essential Fatty Acids
Every fat or oil contains fatty acids, of which eight are known to be essential for the proper functioning of the body. One of the secrets of good nutrition consists in combining these eight E.F.A.s at the same time, since most proteins are deficient in at least one or two of them. Some basic rules for combining specific vegetable proteins

in such a way that a complete usable protein will result are given in Chapter Five.

Carbohydrates

One lifelong student of nutrition who restored many sufferers to health had this to say: 'Too much food improves neither health nor efficiency, but, on the contrary, leads to premature old age and illness.' He was referring particularly to the fact that because of its poor nutritional value over-consumption of food had become a habit amongst the majority of people in the developed parts of the world, especially in the West. These bad habits are further encouraged by debasing taste buds with sugar, synthetic flavourings, salt or other seasoned foods, all in excessive quantities.

As previously stated all white sugar and white flour products have been robbed of most of their nutritive values. The best carbohydrates are found chiefly in wholegrain cereals (including wholemeal flour and brown rice), fresh fruits and vegetables, honey, molasses or dark brown sugar.

CHAPTER FOUR

FOOD SUPPLEMENTS

However carefully food is selected and combined many essential elements may be lacking in these days of growing foods in devitalized or poisoned land and the ever-increasing tendency towards processing and fragmentation. Unless food supplements are taken regularly serious dietary deficiencies may result and these can play a large part in the onset of illnesses such as rheumatism and arthritis.

However, it should be noted that the chemical substitutes obtainable from the chemists bear no relationship to the real thing. For instance, their so-called vitamin C is a substance called ascorbic acid, quite unlike the vitamin C obtainable from the health stores which is derived from rose hips or other naturally growing plants.

It has not yet been established exactly how many vitamins there are but a great deal has been discovered about them.

Vitamin A and Carotene (or Pro-Vitamin A)
Animal foods, particularly fish liver oils, contain vitamin A; vegetable foods, particularly the yellow ones, contain carotene, though some animal foods contain both. If the diet includes nuts, whole cereals such as wholemeal bread, wheat germ, and four to eight dessertspoonsful daily of cod liver oil, there is no danger of a deficiency of these vitamins, and vitamin D will also come into this. Those with arthritis have a special need for these vitamins, and calcium, obtainable at health shops in the form of bone meal, is necessary for their assimilation.

The B Vitamins
The fact that most arthritics have difficulty in assimilating

carbohydrates and consequently can suffer from chronic catarrh may point to a deficiency of the B vitamins. One of the best ways to remedy this is to take brewer's yeast tablets, beginning with two daily, with meals, for three or four weeks, then gradually increasing to six or eight daily. It is generally wise to take about three months before reaching the maximum number, otherwise indigestion may occur, in which case it is best to leave the tablets off altogether for about a week, then go back to two or three. If the body has suffered a deficiency of any specific nutrient over a long period it will not always begin to assimilate it properly over the short term.

Once the system has become used to the brewer's yeast it will be found to help the digestion, and it is also invaluable for the health of the eyes, as I myself have proved on many occasions. However, as well as the yeast it is advisable for those with arthritis to take supplementary vitamin B_{12} (found in liver and in some plants), which is also available in tablet form in health stores. This has been found by experiments to show remarkable results in the treatment of osteo arthritis, though this is not so marked for rheumatoid arthritis. Lean meats (if not overcooked), poultry, fish and milk, dark green leafy vegetables, particularly if eaten raw, nuts and whole grain breads or cereals, all are good sources of various B vitamins. Wheat germ, now freely available in many grocery shops as well as health stores, is rich in most of the B vitamin complex.

Vitamin C
This is contained in many fruits and vegetables, and has been found to be abnormally low in the blood of arthritics. Much has been written about experiments conducted with this vitamin. Everyone suffering from arthritis needs more than normal amounts of vitamin C every day for many reasons too technical to go into here. If it is impracticable to eat large amounts of fruits or vegetables adequate amounts of vitamin C may be obtained from rose hip or other tablets found in health shops. These are

even more effective if combined with the bioflavanoids. The bioflavanoids (vitamin P) occur under the outer skin of citrus fruits.

Most green vegetables, raw or properly cooked in a minimum amount of water or steamed, are excellent sources of vitamin C, as are many fruits.

Vitamin D
This is the so-called sunshine vitamin because it is normally absorbed through the skin in sunny weather and may be in short supply during the winter months or for house-bound people. It is found, like vitamin A, in the fish liver oils, and helps the body to assimilate other substances, particularly calcium. So many vitamins and minerals are more effective when in combination with one another.

Vitamin E
This is particularly useful in cases of muscular rheumatism (fibrositis) and will often give relief when taken in sufficient quantities over a long period of time, even with rheumatic fever and rheumatoid arthritis. Vitamin E plays a large part in assuring that all the cells of the body receive adequate oxygen, the net result being that it increases the flow of blood. It is also useful in counteracting the effects cf rancid or over-processed fats or oils. The recommended quantity to be taken to begin with is two 30 i.u. tablets or capsules twice daily after meals. Later these could be increased to 100 i.u. tablets or capsules, one after each meal. (Incidentally some of these vitamins are stated to be in mg instead of i.u.'s) Each individual must discover by experience the amount he can best tolerate.

Minerals
These are equally important to the health of the body as the vitamins. There are numerous minerals and trace elements required for maximum health but certain substances are so rich in them, balanced and mixed together

in a way in which they can be assimilated by the body, that they deserve special mention.

Wheat Germ
As well as the invaluable vitamin E, wheat germ contains twenty-three known rebuilding minerals.

Sea Vegetables
The most easily obtained sea vegetable is kelp, a seaweed found in deep oceanic waters. It is brought to the land, dried, and can be purchased in powder or tablet form at health food stores. Kelp is one of the best natural sources of iodine, easily digested and assimilated because it is combined with other compatible minerals, vitamins, trace elements, etc. The elements contained in kelp are in the exact proportions needed by the human blood stream. Incidentally, as in the case of the B vitamins, a lack of iodine in the diet can adversely affect the vision.

D. T. Quigley, M.D., has this to say in his book, *The National Malnutrition:* 'Iodine, since it has to do with increasing anti-bacterial elements in the blood, is of value in every type of rheumatic disease.'

Calcium
This is most essential for every cell of the body, particularly for the muscles. A deficiency of calcium can lead to the familiar muscle cramps, and according to Dr L. W. Cromwell in his report to the Gerontological Society of San Francisco, calcium deficiency among his patients has been found to be a cause of arthritic crippling. The regular consumption of bone meal tablets (obtainable at health stores), combined with a healthy diet can help to prevent or eliminate muscle cramp and also to prevent or correct the crumbling or brittleness of the bones (osteoporosis) so often associated with arthritis and with elderly people. This is even more effective when taken in conjunction with wheat germ or vitamin E capsules. It is also more effective when taken along with vitamins A and D. In fact, vitamin D is not well absorbed into the body without it.

Potassium

A mineral of great importance to those suffering from arthritis, since it is an anti-calcification factor and will help to prevent calcium from settling in and stiffening up the joints. This calcification can be caused by a deficiency of either calcium or potassium. Foods rich in potassium are: most green leafy vegetables, celery, wheat germ, kelp, sesame seeds, figs, dark brown sugar (not the dyed variety!), and molasses.

Potassium Broth

Use young carrots with their tops, spinach leaves and stems, chopped-up celery, including leaves, parsley, cabbage and other green vegetables, as available and as fresh as possible. Chop finely, cover with water and simmer gently in a covered saucepan for about thirty minutes. Squeeze out or strain and flavour to taste.

Nuts and Seeds

Nuts and seeds of all kinds are good sources of protein, vitamins, minerals, trace and other elements still unknown to nutritionists. These are so packed with nourishment that they should be used with the greatest moderation. They are expensive (the seeds can be obtained at health stores), but, because of the minimal quantities required, will go far. The most usual ones are sunflower, pumpkin and sesame.

CHAPTER FIVE

MEAT SAVERS AND SUBSTITUTES

It is possible to lead a healthy life by omitting flesh foods entirely from the diet, but in view of the amount of knowledge and experience needed to carry this through successfully, for the great majority of people, particularly the elderly or infirm, any radical or sudden change of diet is not advisable. One particular snag inherent in vegetarianism is that over the long term a vitamin B_{12} deficiency is likely to build up and this can be very serious. To offset this it would be necessary to take regularly tablets of B_{12} obtainable from health stores.

However, replacing flesh foods with vegetarian meals several times weekly would be quite practicable if it is borne in mind that a fully balanced vegetarian meal should contain 'complementary proteins', that is, two or more substances which when combined (and eaten together at the same time) will form a complete protein. Anyone interested in becoming a vegetarian would be advised to obtain books dealing specifically with this subject of complementary proteins, and with vegetarianism in general.

A few recipes using complementary proteins are given below, followed by a table showing other examples of complementary proteins. All complete proteins or complementary protein combinations contain the eight Essential Fatty Acids already referred to in Chapter Three.

Baked Potatoes
If an oven is not available, or seldom used for reasons of

economy, potatoes of a good shape and size may be partially cooked by boiling or steaming, cut in half, and placed under a medium grill for about half an hour. When eaten with cheese this is a complete protein meal.

Spaghetti or Macaroni Bake

This can be left to cook in a preset oven for two hours or a little longer while you are out and then served with a green salad or a green vegetable.

Using one large or two small onions, cut into thin slices lengthwise, stir-fry the onions in two tablespoonsful of butter or margarine until they are transparent and tender – about five minutes. Turn onions into a casserole, spreading them evenly over the bottom. Break 3 oz. (75g) of thin whole wheat spaghetti or macaroni into small pieces and sprinkle them over the onions. Over these put one medium-sized tin of tomatoes, or fresh equivalent, then top with grated cheese, or dot small pieces over all (avoid the processed cheese wrapped in plastic). Cover dish and bake for about two hours in a slow oven 275° to 300°F (135-149°C/Gas Mark 1), according to when you wish it to be ready. This is a complete protein dish.

Rice and Tomato Dish

½ cupful raw brown rice
2 tablespoonsful wheat germ (to complete protein)
1 cupful tomatoes
1 medium onion
sea salt
pepper
½ teaspoonful kelp powder

Bring rice to boil, then cook in fast boiling water until cooked. Slice onion thinly lengthwise and stir-fry until transparent. When the rice is cooked add to it the other ingredients. Put into a shallow dish, sprinkle wholewheat breadcrumbs over the top, dab a little butter on and heat through under a medium grill or in the oven.

The following table gives further examples of complementary proteins:

COMPLEMENTARY VEGETABLE PROTEINS

Complementary Proteins	Proportions
Beans (dried) and any whole grains (whole wheat, oats, etc.).	1 part raw beans to $2\frac{1}{2}$ parts grain.
Dried beans with cheese or other milk product.	1 part raw beans and milk, cheese, etc., according to recipe or to taste.
Dried beans or peas with brown rice.	1 part beans or peas to 4 of cooked rice.
Beans with sesame or sunflower seeds.	1 part beans to 2 of seeds.
Peanut butter or chopped peanuts with dried milk (for sandwiches).	3 parts peanuts to 1 of milk powder.
Peanut butter or peanuts and sunflower seeds (for sandwiches).	Equal quantities.
Potato and milk or milk product, such as cheese.	According to recipe or taste, e.g., baked potato with sprinkle of cheese when split open.
Soy flour with sesame seeds and peanut butter.	Equal quantities. Can be used as a spread (for this the soy flour is roasted until brown in a dry pan and stirred constantly over medium heat).

Small amounts of milk or milk products added to the following can greatly increase the protein quality of the dish: rice, wheat, wheat and peanuts or peanut butter, nuts and seeds, legumes (beans or peas), potatoes. Dried or liquid milk can often be added to the recipes even when this is not called for. If these basic combinations can be borne in mind and followed through when following recipes a food of poor quality can be turned into a good one. For instance, when using baked beans, tinned or home made, milk should be taken at the same meal, or added to the beans, preferably low fat powdered.

A soup made with beans or peas and milk will be a full protein meal. The same will apply if rice or whole wheat flour is used at the same meal. There are many ways of using potatoes with milk products.

Textured Vegetable Proteins

Textured Vegetable Proteins (T.V.P.) are sold under various brand names both in health stores and in some grocery shops. For the most part these food products are based on the soya bean, with certain minerals and vitamins added to make a fully balanced protein food. Blended in with the bean are yeasts, spices and vegetarian flavours which produce meat-like flavours. They are a great deal cheaper than meat or fish and in some ways better, one reason being that they do not produce cholesterol in the body. They will keep indefinitely so long as they remain in the dehydrated state in which they were packaged. They can be bought in various forms, such as minced or chunky.

An analysis of one of the best-known varieties of T.V.P. shows that it contains 52 per cent vegetable protein, a little vegetable fat, and no cholesterol. For arthritics there is the added advantage that unlike many cereals T.V.P. contains no gluten which so many people with arthritis cannot assimilate. This particular T.V.P. (and there is no reason to suppose that other brands are essentially different) also contains the Essential Fatty Acids the body needs as well as many valuable minerals, especially a good proportion of potassium. This mineral is particularly essential for arthritics and is often very deficient in a modern diet. These foods are also fortified with B vitamins, including B_{12}, usually in short supply in vegetarian dishes, but of very vital importance. The calorie content is relatively low compared with the other nutrients.

One word of warning, however; anyone with a goitre or suffering from hypothyroidism, or with a tendency to suffer from a sluggish thyroid or an iodine deficiency should either avoid soya bean products or use them only occasionally. In any case, for all consumers a teaspoonful of kelp (seaweed) powder per person would be a safeguard.

Before using these textured proteins they must be hydrated, i.e., simmered or soaked in water. Directions will be on the packet. Below are a few recipes which can serve as a guide showing different methods of using these proteins to make them appetizing and interesting. There is much room for experimentation, according to the tastes and ingenuity of the user.

Baked Potatoes with T.V.P.

Have ready baked potatoes. Soak or simmer the required amount of minced T.V.P. (about 1 tablespoonful per potato). Cut the potatoes in half and scoop out part of the middle. Mix the T.V.P. with tinned or fresh tomatoes and fill the potato shells with it. Re-heat in oven or under the grill for five to ten minutes.

Another method of using baked potatoes is to stir-fry some thinly-sliced onions, mix these with the T.V.P., and stuff the mixture into the scooped-out potatoes.

A Tasty Meal

Hydrate a small amount of ham or bacon flavoured T.V.P. Mix this into one egg and one tablespoonful of milk which have been beaten well together. Dip required number of slices of wholewheat bread into the mixture and fry both sides (or grill) until golden brown. Alterna-

tively, place in a shallow dish and heat through under a
moderate grill. Tomato ketchup or soya sauce can be used
to flavour if desired.

Savoury Stew

Hydrate ¾ of a teacupful (about 2 oz./50g) of T.V.P.
chunks. Slice two small onions thinly lengthwise and
stir-fry in a little melted butter or margarine until they are
transparent. Add one cupful of tinned or fresh tomatoes,
one tablespoonful brown sugar, a sprinkling of minced
garlic or a crushed clove, a little paprika or chili, along
with some liquid from the tomatoes. Simmer for about
fifteen minutes. Can be served with potatoes and/or green
vegetables.

Baked Beans with T.V.P.

Hydrate ham or bacon flavoured T.V.P. and add to some
heated baked beans, using about one quarter of the
amount of T.V.P. as of the beans. Serve on toast. A little
tomato ketchup or soy sauce may be used if desired.

Soya

Soya flour contains about four times as much protein as
most other cereals and twice as much as pulses. When not
defatted it is about 20 per cent fat. It contains no starch
nor sugar, but is rich in alkaline salts and essential vitamins. In southern China it is almost the only source of
protein in its natural state of the whole bean. Soya flour
can be used to thicken soups, sauces, gravies, etc. One
disadvantage is that it does not keep well and needs to be
used up within two or three months of purchase.

Soya Savoury

Using one tablespoonful of soya flour to three of mashed
potato, blend together. Flavour with onion, chopped
chives, parsley or other herbs and put into a greased pie
dish. Heat through in oven or under grill until slightly
browned.

Soya Milk
Three tablespoonsful of soya flour (preferably defatted) to
$\frac{1}{2}$ pint (275ml) of water. Whisk well together, or put into
blender, and use as milk. If the flour is not defatted it can
be quite rich and should not be consumed in large
quantities nor with great frequency.

Soya Cheese
One quart (1 litre) of soya milk. Bring this to the boil. As
it begins to rise, pour in three quarters of a tablespoonful
of fresh lemon juice. Let stand until cold. Then strain
through muslin, squeeze out all moisture and use as
cottage cheese. Flavour to taste.

Whey – the liquid whey remaining after the making of
the cheese – is a very valuable food. (If ordinary milk is
used instead of a soya milk, cottage cheese can be made
by using the above method.) The whey is the plasma part
of the milk, i.e., the milk modified by the lactic acid
culture. It contains much of the sugar and salts of the milk
and also has an antibiotic reaction.

A small amount of soya flour added to breads, cakes,
pastries or other cereal foods can greatly improve their
food value.

Legumes (Dried Beans, Peas, Lentils, Peanuts)
These are all deficient in one or two of the essential amino
acids which the body needs to make up a complete usable
protein. The table on page 27 lists complementary foods
which can be added to make up the deficiencies.

All proteins should be consumed in very moderate
amounts by those with arthritis. I think it is safe to say, for
instance, that three or four tablespoonsful of dried
legumes, will be ample at any one meal for anyone getting
on in years or unable for any reason to take a lot of
strenuous physical exercise. Legumes of any sort are apt
to be 'clogging' foods when used too frequently or in large
helpings at a time. Those with arthritis would be well
advised to use them only once or at most twice weekly. If
surplus amounts are soaked and cooked they can be put

into the freezer or freezing compartment of the refrigerator for future use. Some sample recipes follow:

Bean Stew with Dumplings
(This combination provides a complete usable protein)
  1 small cupful beans (soaked overnight)
  1 medium onion
  1 small parsnip (optional)
  1 teaspoonful cooking oil or fat
  2 small carrots
  vegetable stock

Slice onions lengthwise and brown in fat. Add to a cupful of vegetable stock. Scrub carrots and cut into thin rings; cut parsnip into three or four strips lengthwise, then into inch-long pieces. Add the vegetables to stock mixture and simmer until the beans are soft, adding extra water or stock as necessary. Add vegetable or yeast extract for flavour. *Dumplings* (to be added during last half hour of cooking): Take one cupful (approx. 6 oz./175g) of wholemeal, self-raising flour and rub in one tablespoonful butter or margarine. Moisten sufficiently with cold water so that the dough can be shaped into small balls. Drop these into the stewing pan, cover, and simmer for about one-half hour.

Bean Loaf
Put cooked haricot or other beans through a meat grinder, sieve, or blender with a little liquid, or mash them. Add one quarter the amount of grated cheese, a little grated onion, and enough whole wheat breadcrumbs to make the mixture into a loaf. Season to taste. Bake in a moderate oven, basting occasionally with a little fat. This may also be put into a shallow dish and heated through under a moderate grill.

Vegetable Casserole
  ¼ cupful dried beans – pre-soaked and cooked
  ¼ lb (100g) fresh green beans, sliced thinly

½ teaspoonful chili powder (or less: this is very strong)
1 cupful tinned or frozen corn kernels
2 tablespoonsful grated cheese
½ cupful sliced tomatoes, fresh or tinned
a little salt
soya sauce

Mix together the cooked beans, corn kernels, soy sauce, and other seasonings. Into a greased casserole place alternate layers of these and the other ingredients, adding cheese last. Bake in a moderate oven for about thirty minutes. Basil and sage (sprinklings only) may be added instead of chili if preferred. Beans and cheese make up complementary protein. (Soya sauce is available in most grocery shops.)

Bean Meal
1 cupful haricot or kidney beans, soaked overnight

Using the water in which the beans were soaking, add one medium sliced onion, one medium sliced carrot, a crushed garlic clove or a sprinkle of minced dried garlic (sold in jars), one teaspoonful sea salt, one teaspoonful thyme. Let all these cook together over a low heat until the beans are tender. This will be one and a half to two hours, depending on the beans. While the mixture is still hot, stir in two tablespoonsful desiccated coconut which has been well blended with a little milk or cream.

While the bean mixture is cooking prepare and cook brown rice or potatoes to go with it. If potatoes are used they should be mashed, using a little milk. Either rice or milk-potatoes will make a complementary protein with the beans.

CHAPTER SIX

MEAT AND FISH DISHES

It is generally accepted that both meat and fish are acid-producing, so that the wise course for arthritics would be to use them no more than once each day, and then in small or moderate helpings. There is also the consideration that much of the meat sold today comes from animals which can harbour residues such as hormones, antibiotics and other substances which can be harmful over the long term. This would apply particularly to animals or birds raised in confined spaces, such as calves, pigs and battery hens.

Fish is more easily digested than meat and less likely to be contaminated. It is also a good source of vitamins A and D, which are so important for arthritics.

Liver and Apples
  4 slices liver
  1½ tablespoonsful melted butter
  1 small tart apple, sliced and peeled
  1 tablespoonful wheat germ
  pinch of powdered thyme
  sea salt to taste

Mix together thyme, salt and wheat germ. Dip liver in the melted butter and sprinkle over it the wheat germ mixture. Brown in the fat on both sides. Leave in pan and cover with the apple. Cover and cook over low heat for about fifteen minutes. Liver is a good source of minerals and B vitamins.
(The above recipe is reproduced courtesy of Prevention *magazine.)*

Baked Chicken Legs
  2 chicken legs
  2 slices bacon

1 small carrot
1 small onion (thinly sliced)
1 tablespoonful sherry
1 cupful vegetable or other stock
a pinch of mixed herbs
sea salt and pepper

Remove meat from the legs and put it with the bacon into a thick-bottomed saucepan. Add the rest of the ingredients except the sherry and simmer until the meat is tender. Add the sherry and serve.

Lamb or Mutton Stew
1 lb (450g) neck or breast of meat
1 medium onion, cut thinly
3 medium potatoes
2 or 3 medium tomatoes
2 or 3 large slices of vegetable marrow
3 tablespoonsful raw rice
salt and pepper

Remove skin and superfluous fat from the meat and cut it into small pieces. Put it into a saucepan, cover with water and bring it slowly to the boil. Remove scum, add the vegetables and again bring to the boil. Cover the pan and simmer very gently for about half an hour, then sprinkle in the rice and cook slowly for another half hour, or until the meat and rice are cooked.

Sweet and Sour Beef
2 cupsful cooked beef (cut into cubes)
1 tablespoonful melted butter
2 tablespoonsful flour
1 onion, cut into thin strips
$\frac{1}{2}$ cupful brown sugar
$\frac{1}{2}$ teaspoonful dry mustard
3 tablespoonsful of cider-apple vinegar
cooked rice, preferably brown

Stir-fry the onions in the hot fat until they are transparent. Brown the meat slightly. Remove both from pan. Mix the

flour into a paste with a little cold water. Add a little more
water and turn into frying pan. Stir constantly until
brown, adding more fat if necessary. Put all ingredients
into a saucepan, cover with water and simmer for about
half an hour. To serve pour over hot fluffy rice. Less meat
may be used, in which case it would be necessary to vary
quantities of other ingredients accordingly.

Cooked Cod or Haddock with Cheese
About $\frac{1}{2}$ lb (225g) or less of cooked fish (broken into
    flakes). Remove skin and bones
2 tablespoonsful butter
2-3 tablespoonsful grated cheese
$\frac{1}{4}$ cupful water
1 tablespoonful flour
1 cupful milk
breadcrumbs
salt and pepper

Melt the butter in a saucepan, add the flour and blend
well. Stir in the water, bring to the boil, stirring constantly. Simmer for five minutes. Add the milk, fish,
cheese and seasoning. Turn the mixture into a shallow
pan or dish which will go under the grill. Cover with fine
breadcrumbs, scatter a few pieces of butter or margarine
over the top and brown under a medium grill, watching to
see that it does not burn or dry up. Salmon or other white
fish can also be cooked in this way.

Steamed Fish
1 medium potato per person
1 medium carrot per person
fish fillets, fresh or frozen
peas
medium onion
salt and pepper

Peel potato and cut it into thin slices. Cut carrots into thin
rounds. Cook potatoes and carrots together in just enough

water to cover, add peas. Cut onion lengthwise into thin slices, stir-fry in a little butter.

When the onions are almost soft, set them with the fish in a pan or plate on top of the saucepan containing the potatoes and other vegetables, or other vessel containing boiling water.

Prepare Tomato-Soya Sauce (see Sauce section, p. 38) and pour it over the fish and onions.

Creamed Fish
Left-over cooked fish may be heated between two plates over steam, then served with brown sauce, plain or with parsley or other herbs. See also Sauce section for ideas.

Fish Cakes
Use remnants of any cooked fish with skin and bones removed. Mix this with mashed potato and a little milk into a stiff consistency. Add salt and pepper and a little chopped parsley. Form the mixture into cakes and brown in hot fat. Any surplus can be wrapped in grease-proof paper and put into freezer or freezing compartment until wanted.

N.B. A little onion which has been cooked by stir-frying will add zest to any steamed or boiled fish or meat. Stir-frying is a Chinese way of cooking which retains all the goodness of the vegetables. It means using a medium heat and stirring the vegetables constantly in enough fat to coat them to the point where they are crisp and their flavour is at its height. They should not taste raw and they should not be brown.

CHAPTER SEVEN

SAUCES AND MARINADES

Tomato Sauce
    1 cupful of chopped tomatoes, fresh or tinned
    1 small onion
    2 tablespoonsful melted butter or margarine
    1 teaspoonful of bayleaf powder
    1 dessertspoonful of cider vinegar
    1 tablespoonful flour
    sea salt and pepper to taste

Put the finely-sliced or chopped onion and all the other ingredients except the flour and butter into a saucepan and boil till tender. Rub the mixture through a sieve. Stir the flour into the melted fat, add a little milk or water and bring to boil, stirring constantly. Add the tomato mixture very gradually and bring to boil, stirring all the time.

Quick Tomato-Soya Sauce
One dessertspoonful whole wheat flour or semolina to half a cupful of water or milk. If flour is used mix this with a little of the liquid into a smooth paste, add the remainder of the liquid and heat to boiling point over a medium fire, stirring constantly. For semolina sprinkle this over the water or milk and bring to boil, stirring all the time. If the mixture is too thick a little milk can be added as it heats. When the right consistency is reached add one table-spoonful of tomato ketchup and one teaspoonful of soya sauce.

Brown Sauce Helene
    1 small teaspoonful dry mustard
    1 large tablespoonful brown sugar

2 teaspoonsful cider vinegar
1 tablespoonful flour
1 cupful of water
handful of sultanas
little stewed apple
sprinkling of powdered bay leaf
sea salt

Mix well together all dry ingredients (not the fruit, which can be optional). To these add the vinegar and water, and fruit, if used. Bring slowly to boil, stirring all the time until slightly thickened. Use for gammon or fish.

Curry Sauce
2 oz. (50g) butter or margarine
2 tablespoonsful flour
1 cupful cold milk or water
1 to 3 tablespoonsful curry powder (according to taste)
2 tablespoonsful tomato ketchup
2 tablespoonsful desiccated coconut
1 small onion, chopped finely
2 tablespoonsful chopped chutney
1 finely chopped apple (peeled and cored)
2 or 3 tablespoonsful soaked sultanas (optional)
a pinch of cayenne pepper
$\frac{1}{2}$ clove garlic

Heat the onions in the melted fat over a medium heat, stirring constantly until transparent. Add the curry powder, stirring well in. Mix the flour into a smooth paste with a little of the cold milk or water, add this alternately with the rest of the liquid to the fat-onion-curry mixture, blending well together over a slow heat. Stir in the tomato ketchup. Add chutney, chopped apple and coconut and other ingredients if used. Simmer slowly over a low heat for about fifteen minutes, stirring frequently.

Any surplus sauce can be stored in a covered jar in the refrigerator for two to four days, and thinned down with cold milk or water before re-heating if necessary.

Tartare Sauce
Put into a bowl a tablespoonful each of Worcester Sauce
and cider vinegar, a tablespoonful of lemon juice, a little
salt and one to two cupsful of water (according to taste
and amount required). Set the bowl into a pan of hot
water to heat the ingredients through.

Black Butter Sauce
   4 tablespoonsful of butter or margarine
   1 dessertspoonful of cider vinegar
   1 dessertspoonful chopped parsley
   salt and pepper

Brown oil in the saucepan and when it has cooled slightly
add the vinegar, then re-heat very slowly but do not boil.
Add parsley and seasoning.

Marinades
Marinades are useful for softening tough meats or im-
parting flavour to uninteresting fish. These can be soaked
in the marinade for about half an hour before being
cooked.

Simple Marinade
This is made in the proportion of two tablespoonsful of
vegetable oil to one of cider vinegar or lemon juice, to
which can be added chopped parsley or other herbs,
chopped onions or chives. Red or white wine and a little
redcurrant jelly can also be added. Scores can be made in
the meat or fish before putting it into the marinade.

CHAPTER EIGHT

SALADS, SOUPS AND SANDWICHES

A good salad can provide a well-balanced and highly palatable meal, given a little forethought and imagination, and it need not be expensive, even in winter time. The variations are infinite. However, for those not used to eating raw foods it is wise to begin with to avoid too many mixtures. Start with about one teaspoonful of one raw green vegetable, perhaps parsley, and combine it with baked or steamed potato. After a few days another raw food could be added, say a little grated carrot. In all cases salads must be very thoroughly masticated if they are to be properly digested and they should never be eaten in a hurry.

Lettuce may be used with the leaves whole or shredded. Raw cabbage is a good substitute for lettuce, which is so often priced above its food value in the shops. Cabbage is fairly easy to digest if it is finely chopped or grated and eaten in small quantities at a time.

Suggested Combinations for Salads
Orange, dates, and nuts (only one or two nuts per person)
Orange, dates and sunflower or pumpkin seeds
Raw, chopped apple with two or three nuts, lettuce and cucumber
Celery, apple, nuts or seeds, with cheese
Pineapple and cream or cottage cheese
Raw carrot with sultanas, apple and dates
Raw carrot with sultanas and bananas
Raw carrot and raw cabbage with sultanas and dates

These are only a few of the many combinations which can be used to make salads which are palatable, nutritious, and easily put together. Any of these could be served with cottage cheese, which is an excellent protein food.

A Basic Salad Dressing

Three tablespoonsful of olive or other vegetable oil to a tablespoonful of cider vinegar. Mix together and add two teaspoonsful of brown sugar. Shake well (best done in a jar) and add a tablespoonful of milk.

This dressing will keep indefinitely. The proportions can be altered according to taste.

Soups

Properly made and well-balanced soups can be a great standby, and can often be a meal in themselves, particularly in times of unusual stress, or when one is suffering from colds or other minor ailments, or recovering from more serious setbacks. They are a special boon to the elderly and others who are alone or handicapped. Any soup left over from the whole recipe can be stored for two or three days in a jar in the refrigerator. This is a saving on time, energy, and fuel. A good vegetable stock can be used as a base for many soups.

Vegetable Stock

 1 cupful carrots, shredded or diced
 1 cupful celery, leaves and all, finely diced
 1 cupful any other vegetable or vegetables (beet tops, turnip tops, and parsley are particularly nutritious)

This stock can in fact be made with whatever vegetables are available, in any combinations, both roots and tops. It can be flavoured with herbs such as marjoram, bay leaves, thyme, tied together with cotton or put into a muslin bag so that they can be withdrawn when the soup is ready for the table.

Using, if available, a stainless steel or enamel rather than an aluminium pan, put in the vegetables and add water to cover and an inch or two more. Put on lid and cook slowly for about half an hour. Strain, squeeze juice from the pulp and store in the refrigerator or cold larder and amount not being used immediately.

Legume Soups

All bean or pea (legume) soups if eaten with cheese or

milk will provide a complete protein dish. Legumes and rice (preferably brown), a tablespoonful of wheat germ or unprocessed wheat bran to a serving, accompanied by whole wheat bread will provide a well-balanced protein meal. Sesame or sunflower seeds when eaten at the same meal as legumes also make a complete protein, equal in quality to beef steak.

The following is a useful guide for compatible herbs and vegetables:

For celery soup – nutmeg or dill

For pulses (lentils, split peas, etc.) – rosemary, marjoram, mint, parsley, thyme

For onion soups – sage

For potato soup – chives, mint, parsley, caraway seeds,
   nutmeg

For tomato soup – basil, marjoram, chives, mace

Quick Lentil Soup
Precook half a cupful of dry lentils

   1 small onion, cut into thin lengthwise strips
   1 carrot, cut into thin lengthwise strips

Brown the onions and carrots in a small amount of vegetable oil or butter, then add a little thyme and/or marjoram.

   1½ cupsful of vegetable stock or water seasoned with a
      little Marmite and soy sauce
   ½ cupful of tomatoes, fresh or tinned
   salt and pepper to taste

Heat all the above ingredients together, then add a little chopped parsley, and if desired two or three tablespoon-fuls of sherry. If grated cheese (about two tablespoonsful per person) is added to the soup you have a full protein meal.

Cream of Bean Soup
Using tinned baked beans, put these through a sieve or liquidizer-blender with a little water added. Turn into a

saucepan and heat through slowly, adding a little milk at a time to required amount, but not allowing it to boil. This can be served with buttered whole wheat toast.

Dumplings
Dumplings added to vegetable soups will in many cases make a 'complete' protein and produce a better balanced meal. This can be an alternative to whole wheat bread or toast.

Basic Dumpling Recipe
One and a half cupsful of whole wheat flour to two level tablespoonsful of vegetable fat and a teaspoonful of baking powder and a little salt.

Rub fat well into the flour until the mixture is of breadcrumb consistency. Add herbs, if desired, and enough water to make a soft but not too sticky dough. Flour hands well and form the doughdough into small balls. Drop them into the simmering soup or hot water half an hour before serving.

Sandwiches and Spreads
My study of articles on nutrition and my own personal experience convince me that all cereal products should be consumed in moderate quantities by those suffering from arthritis, bread, preferably whole wheat, being limited to two or three rounds daily. One of the reasons for this is that, with few exceptions (rice, I believe being one), all cereals contain gluten, which many arthritics have difficulty in assimilating. Another is, of course, the likelihood of obesity if they are eaten in large quantities, when they also inhibit the appetite for the more healing foods such as fruits and vegetables. The following suggestions might be useful for special occasions.

Peanut Butter
By itself this is not a complete usable protein. To make a completely usable protein sandwich use whole wheat bread and one of the following combinations:

Peanut butter mixed with just under one part of dried skim milk to two of the peanut butter.

Mashed banana can be added to the above, along with a little sharp-tasting jelly, such as red-currant. Spread on top of the peanut butter mixture it gives it a pleasant tang.

As above, without the mashed banana.

Two parts of the peanut butter to one of wheat germ instead of powdered milk.

Split a banana in half, lengthwise. Mix peanut butter with powdered milk and spread this over one half. Put the two parts together again, dip into orange juice and roll in wheat germ. This makes a well-balanced protein meal.

Peanut butter with chopped dates, mashed banana and a little wheat germ or powdered milk.

As above with a little mashed avocado pear.

Peanut butter with cottage cheese is a good protein.

CHAPTER NINE

DESSERTS AND CONFECTIONS

Stewed Apples with Dates
This recipe will use half a pound (225g) of cooking apples to a handful of dates, with a little water. Cook prepared apples and dates together very slowly in the water until the apples are fluffy. Serve hot or cold with cream or yogurt.
    When cool this can be made more interesting by folding into it egg white beaten stiff or whipped cream.

Alternatively, after cooking, pour into a shallow dish or pan, top with wheat germ or a little quick oats, a few dabs of butter and a little dark brown sugar. Heat this under a low grill for ten to fifteen minutes. Cornflakes or other dry cereal can also be used for topping.

Yogurt Compote

To a cupful of yogurt and a dessertspoonful of honey, blended well together, add three tablespoonsful desiccated coconut, half a cupful of soaked dried apricots or sliced fresh ones, half a cupful of grated apple, a little almond extract, and two or three tablespoonsful of chopped or ground nuts.

This is quick and easy to prepare and useful in suitable quantities for unexpected guests.

Quick Crust

   2 cupsful granola
   $\frac{1}{2}$ cupful whole wheat flour
   2 tablespoonsful powdered milk
   $\frac{1}{4}$ cupful cooking oil or melted margarine

Mix dry ingredients together and stir the oil well in, very gradually, making sure the mixture does not become too moist. Spread over the bottom of a pie dish and put filling on top, or in the case of a fruit pie spread the granola crust on top. Heat through in a moderate oven or under a moderate grill.

Cheese Crust

Mix together half a cupful of mild cheese (grated) and a cupful of whole wheat flour (or if preferred half a cupful each of whole wheat and white flour). Add half a teaspoonful of salt. Drop in about a tablespoonful of water and stir or cut this into the mixture until it is all blended, adding a little more water drop by drop if necessary. When the mixture can be handled roll it out on a floured board and use as desired.

Crispy Porcupines
  1 egg
  ½ cupful brown sugar
  1 teaspoonful vanilla essence
  3 cupsful puffed wheat or rice previously crisped in oven or under grill if they have gone limp
  desiccated coconut
  1½ cupsful chopped dates
  2 tablespoonsful melted butter or margarine or cooking oil

Combine beaten egg, sugar, dates and vanilla. Cook for about fifteen minutes over medium heat, stirring constantly to prevent sticking. Cool slightly, then add oil and puffed rice or wheat. Mix well. Shape into small balls. Sprinkle the coconut on to a board and roll the balls in it. These sweets will keep indefinitely in the freezing compartment or freezer.

No-Bake Fruit Bars
  1 cupful seedless raisins
  1 cupful assorted dried fruit
  ¼ cupful digestive or other biscuit crumbs
  ½ cupful almonds
  ¼ cupful dried milk powder
  3-4 tablespoonsful molasses
  desiccated coconut (optional)

Chop fruit and nuts. Combine with milk powder and biscuit crumbs, then add molasses very gradually and mix well. Shape into logs about an inch round and long enough to handle with ease. (These will be easier to handle if rolled in coconut or ground nuts.) Wrap in foil or a plastic bag to store or slice into one inch bars and serve immediately. Will keep best in freezing compartment or deep freezer.
(The above recipe is reproduced courtesy of Prevention magazine.)

Wheat Germ Sweet
One tablespoonful of black molasses, a teaspoonful of

honey heated together in a bowl set over hot water. Add half a cupful of dry skim milk powder and a cupful of wheat germ. Knead together on board, adding ground nuts or nuts cut into small pieces. Form into small pieces and roll in ground nuts. These snacks are packed full of good nourishment and can be kept indefinitely in a freezing compartment or deep freezer. If desired desiccated coconut may be used in place of the ground nuts to roll the balls in.

A SUMMING-UP

If the whole of this book were summarized in a few words, what would emerge would be something along these lines:

1. Everyone with arthritis should be more concerned with quality rather than quantity of food.
2. The right kinds of food eaten in moderate quantities will not produce obesity which is so often one of the greatest handicaps for those attempting to cope with arthritis in any of its forms.
3. White flour and white sugar products should be consumed in very limited quantities.
4. It is helpful to eat a little fresh fruit or raw salad *before* each meal.
5. Proteins of any sort should be consumed sparingly.
6. The bulk of the diet should consist of vegetables (raw or cooked), including potatoes cooked in their jackets, fruits, moderate quantities of whole cereals, some protein foods, including nuts and seeds, such as sunflower. Nuts and seeds are valuable sources of trace elements, as well as vitamins, minerals and protein.